~JUICING~

The Secret to Anti-Aging, Longevity, Vitality & Weight Loss

By
Dr. Linda Marquez Goodine, D.C.

Printed in the United States of America

Juicing: The Secret To Anti-Aging, Longevity,
Vitality & Weight Loss

ISBN: 978-0-9899351-0-4

Cover Design By:
Lynn M. Snyder
Nosy Rosy Designs
nosyrosydesigns@gmail.com

Page Layout By:
Patt Davis
PD Partners Consulting
www.pattdavis.com

DEDICATION

This book is dedicated to my high school sweetheart, my best friend, the love of my life and husband David for his unconditional support and encouragement. And to my amazing children Cassandra, Trenton and Monet for being the best children in the world because without you I wouldn't have the drive to do this.

My parents who I know are the best parents in the world for their endless love and support in my triumphs and challenges through this journey called life. My special childhood BFF Zonia Aguilar for your help in all the little things you do that make a big difference. Dr. Tony Ganem, your endless support, abundant opportunities and commitment that taught me to be the best practitioner I could be to serve mankind. My amazing friend and coach Kimberly Rinaldi, who helped remove my limiting beliefs by saying "K.T.S.O.", in her kind and loving ways and Ruben Mata your endless encouragement. And last but not least none of this would be possible without God, who gave me the gifts and talents to be who I am today. I know that "All Things Are Possible With God".

DISCLAIMER NOTICE

The author's purpose of this book is to educate and encourage positive changes for extraordinary health. The author or publisher does not guarantee that anyone following the techniques, suggestions, tips, ideas, or strategies will become successful.

The suggestions in this book are not intended as a substitute for proper medical advice. Always consult your physician or healthcare professional, before implementing any new physical activity or dietary changes, especially if you're pregnant or nursing, elderly, have chronic or recurring conditions.

The author and publisher do not warrant that the information contained in this book is fully complete and shall not be responsible for any errors or omissions or for any special or consequential damage caused or alleged to be caused directly or indirectly by the information contained in this book. Any duplication or redistribution of this product without written consent from the author is strictly prohibited.

Table of Contents

Introduction 1

Chapter 1 - Where's your health 3

Chapter 2 - The foundation for a healthy diet 13

Chapter 3 - Why should I juice? 27

Chapter 4 - What should I expect from juicing? 35

Chapter 5 - What is the difference between juice
fasting, blending and adding juicing to my current
dietary regime? 39

Chapter 6 - Steps for getting started! 41

Chapter 7 - Taking action for a juice fast and
permanent lifestyle changes 55

Chapter 8 - Getting the most out of a juice fast 63

Chapter 9 - Juice recipes for extraordinary health 75

Chapter 10 - Blended smoothies, blended soups and
blended drinks 97

Chapter 11 - Q & A: Quick answers to your juicing
questions 111

Appendix A 117

Appendix B 118

Notes 119

INTRODUCTION

Congratulations on taking a step toward a new and healthier you. This is the right time for you to implement the information in this book. If you were not interested in achieving greater health you wouldn't be reading this book now.

Juicing has become a way of life for me after struggling for years with my energy level, gaining and losing weight and always on a diet. I have been studying health, nutrition and fitness for over 30 years and have tried about every diet, weight loss supplement, and program that promises an amazing body and energy in a matter of days. What I have discovered after years of trial and error are the little gems of information that you will be able to apply to your life if you are looking for a path that will keep you young, energetic and slim.

You will be learning a lot of information but it's not a comprehensive book. This book has been written to have you take immediate action. It has been written for people who are very busy, don't have a lot of time to read and want the nuts and bolts of achieving great health.

I encounter people almost on a daily basis who talk about how horrible they feel, how they wish they could shed a few extra pounds, how they lack energy, how quickly they are aging; and they blame it on genetics, their work or family life but will never take the first step to make a change. They will always talk about the problem and seldom talk about the solution. I always say if they exerted the same amount of effort into finding solutions and applying them, as they do into destroying their health and complaining about it they wouldn't be where they are now.

I can relate to this, because I have done it myself. Why do we keep on doing the same thing and expecting different results? Some have defined this as insanity. I would have to agree because I have been there. I remember the wasted time and energy spent on complaining about the problem and not focusing on the solution.

Consider this a step, whether it's your first step or the one hundredth step on your journey to achieving great health, extraordinary energy and an amazingly fit body. This book will change your health and your life. I hope that you will find the information in this book as exciting as I did in writing it.

You will find some pages that allow you to take notes or apply an action step, so that you can reach your desired health goals. It's time to move toward the solution instead of focusing on the problem. I highly recommend you read this book in its entirety before starting a juice fast or if you will be supplementing your daily routine with juicing.

~JUICING~

The Secret to Anti-Aging, Longevity, Vitality and Weight Loss

CHAPTER 1

Where's Your Health?

In America we are suffering from a major health crisis. Every day we hear about the war on cancer and the increasing number of people who have become victims of heart disease, and diabetes, not to mention the obesity epidemic in America.

Most Diseases Are Preventable

Did you know that according to the CDC[1], 7 out of 10 deaths in the U.S. are from chronic diseases? Heart disease, stroke and cancer account for more than 50% of all deaths that occur each year.[2] These diseases are preventable with lifestyle changes. The most common and costly of these diseases are:

- Heart disease
- Cancer
- Stroke
- Diabetes
- Arthritis

Is anyone noticing that more people are being killed by conventional medicine mistakes?[3] What about the half million Americans dying every year from modern medicine[4]?

- Approximately 783,000 people die every year from conventional medicine
- Over 1 million patients are injured in U.S. hospitals each year
- Approximately 280,000 die annually from injuries in hospitals
- Over 100,000 people a year die from prescription drugs

Do you want to become a statistic? I don't think so. Otherwise you wouldn't be taking action right now to change your health. Don't leave your health in the hands of someone else.

Why Is The U.S. Failing When It Comes To Great Health and Longevity?

It's interesting how we are considered one of the super powers of the world; with some of the best health care facilities in the world but we also have the highest infant mortality rate and the lowest life expectancy. The U.S. spends more on health care than any other industrialized nation in the world and we are still one of the unhealthiest in the world. I would have to use the word *healthcare* loosely and insert the word *sick care*.

Where Is Your Health?

It is interesting that currently over 44 million Americans are without health insurance and 38 million have inadequate health insurance.[5]

Americans also spend 17.9 % of GDP (gross domestic product), the highest in the world on health care expenditures.[6]

Your Sickness is Big Money

Sickness is a big business and the pharmaceutical companies know this. "Big Pharma" has deep pockets that support politicians who will allow them to buy many favors. I also believe insurance companies are for profit and so they continue to increase their premiums to put more money in their pockets. Their primary objective is making profits versus delivering quality healthcare. The bottom line is that sickness is a big business. Why would your doctor want you to get healthy at the expense of his/her pocket book? I am not saying that all doctors' main objective is to prioritize making money over providing excellent health care to their patients. I believe some physicians have their hands tied while trying to provide quality care as proficient, competent, and caring physicians, because of the limitations set upon them by the insurance companies.

With all that said, aren't you glad you made a decision to start taking responsibility for your health? I'm sure glad that you did!

Why Are We So Unhealthy?

Most people think that if they could lose weight they would get healthy. If that were the case, what happens to the person who undergoes liposuction or has gastric banding, sheds 20 pounds and continues the same lifestyle, would that make them healthy? Of course not because what caused the initial problems was never addressed! Most healthy people are not overweight but most overweight people are unhealthy.

According to the World Health Organization, the definition of *health is,* ***"Health is a state of complete physical, mental and social well-being and not merely the absence of disease or infirmity."*** This I find interesting because many people tell me, "I feel fine and I'm as healthy as a horse." But the following week, we are attending the funeral of the so called "I'm healthy as a horse" person, after they died from a massive heart attack. I should have asked what kind of horse they were. You get my point. We can't equate our health with the absence of symptoms. By the time your symptoms show up, the disease process has been developing for some time. Most people will ignore the symptoms of headaches, pain, constipation, diarrhea, allergies, fatigue, PMS, foggy brain, sleep disturbances, skin disorders, emotional instability, and **weight gain** as a warning sign that their body is malfunctioning.

Where Is Your Health?

They have been accustomed to *taking a pill* to mask the symptoms. This is as ridiculous as spray-painting the dash board on your car when the "check engine light" or "service engine soon light" goes on. Most of us would schedule an appointment with our mechanic to get the vehicle checked, find out the cause of the problem and get it fixed. Why don't we do that with our own bodies? It's crazy!!! Our body is our vehicle for life as it takes us to work, the beach, the grocery store, on hikes and long walks while visiting our favorite vacationing spot!

Most people, especially Americans, will rely on a drug to take away the symptoms. In America it has become the norm to fix the problem the quickest way possible because we have become a "fast food" society and many have applied this to their health by taking a pill. Unfortunately it's the same medication that they took for their original problem that will usually create other health issues like constipation, liver toxicity, fatigue, pain and sleep issues.

The most common symptom of unhealthiness is being overweight. Obesity and many other health conditions are primarily due to blood sugar issues and chemical toxicity. We have become a nation that eats everything but real food. The majority of the food we eat is chemically processed, loaded with sugar, preservatives and genetically modified organisms, which leads to disease and hormonal imbalance in body. I believe it's the chemicals that have created an epidemic of sickness and obesity.

Although the subject of this book is juicing, I need to lay some groundwork, so that I accomplish my mission of getting you to start juicing, making permanent lifestyle changes, and looking and feeling amazing! You may be thinking, "Okay, she said that just because we may not feel any symptoms, that doesn't equate to health," right? That is true. I always recommend that clients consult with their physician prior to starting any exercise program or making changes to their diet when they have a health condition.

How Do You Know You Are Healthy?

Some of the recommendations I make with my clients are: a physical exam, comprehensive blood tests and relevant diagnostic tests be performed prior to starting their journey to health. It should be done for 2 reasons:

1. Know the status of your current health
2. Have a baseline of 6 months for comparison

Unfortunately most people don't have screening tests done due to a lack of finances, don't know which tests they need, or their doctor is limited by the insurance company as to what test are allowed to be run. Well let's look at the first reason, lack of finances. It always costs less to floss and brush your teeth than it does to get a root canal done.

I remember a client that complained about a toothache for years and I advised him to go to the dentist for a check up but he stated that he didn't have a couple of hundred dollars to get the dental work done but was going to purchase a new cell phone. A couple of months later, after having suffered for a year, he informed me that he had a tooth abscess that had spread to his other teeth and the cost was going to be in the thousands of dollars compared to the couple of hundred it would have cost if he would have taken care of the it at the initial signs of the problem.

The moral of the story is: it costs more to fix something than to maintain it. Just because you don't have pain or symptoms it doesn't necessarily mean you are healthy. Since we get 6 months dental checkups and I think we should also get blood tests done every 6 months, to see if our health is progressing or regressing, which brings me to my 2nd point. Get blood tests done every 6 months so that you have a baseline and can compare your test results to see if your health is moving in the right direction. Trust me on this one! This is from personal experience. I looked like the picture of health but was tired most of the time, which I attributed to my schedule (who wouldn't be with a schedule like mine). I was actually dying and going down quickly. It wasn't until I had blood tests and hormone testing done that I was able to get some answers and turn my health around.

Remember the definition of health?

"Health is a state of complete physical, mental and social well-being and not merely the absence of disease or infirmity."

How's Your Physical Health?

I think one of the best ways to determine our health is by looking in the mirror naked! Some of you may be frightened by the idea. The mirror doesn't lie and has been true and tested. I often think of a mirror like talking to kids, they tell the truth about what they see and they don't hesitate about giving you an honest answer that may hurt your feelings.

Look at your muscle tone.
      - Is it flabby? Or is it firm and toned?
Look at your hair.
      - Is it lifeless? Is it falling out? Or is it
        thick and shiny?
Look at your eyes.
      - Are they watery, itchy and red? Or are
        they sparkling?

Where Is Your Health?

Look at your skin.
> - Is it full of blemishes, reddish and speckled with brown spots? Or is unblemished, smooth and radiant.

Look at your nails.
> - Are they brittle, have ridges, have a brown band, and look like they are scooped out? Or are they strong, smooth and pinkish in color?

Look at your tongue.
> - Is it swollen, inflamed, have a white coating or bright red? Or is it light to medium pink in color?

Do you find yourself huffing and puffing after climbing a flight of stairs? How do you feel after chasing your little one around the house? After a few minutes are you exhausted and out of breath? Do you find yourself spending more time sleeping throughout the day instead of spending time outdoors or enjoying hobbies with friends and family?

If you are suffering from fatigue, pain, sleep issues or any other symptoms, your body is giving you a warning sign; something is wrong and warrants further investigation. A person without symptoms doesn't necessarily warrant a healthy body either. One of the best indicators of good health is appearance, energy, negative test results and the ability to handle stress in a positive manner. *"Health is a state of complete physical, mental and social well-being and not merely the absence of disease or infirmity."*

~JUICING~

CHAPTER 2

The Foundation For A Healthy Diet

1. Water – "Elixir For Life"

Your body is made of approximately 60% water. Water helps maintain a balance of your body's fluids. Keeping up your body's fluid levels is important for digestion, elimination, regulating body temperature, nutrient absorption and the production of saliva. I also believe it helps to detoxify your body. When you spill something on the driveway, what do you do? You wash it off with water right? Have you heard the expression "dilute the pollution"?

Are You Hungry or Thirsty?

Staying hydrated helps curb your appetite because it makes you feel full. Most of the time we mistake hunger for thirst and eat sugary foods for quick energy or drink high caloric beverages like soft drinks. The next time you feel hungry grab a glass of water or opt for vegetables with high water content.

Beauty Drink

Water is also a beauty drink and is great for your skin. When you are dehydrated your skin appears more dry and wrinkled. What's the difference between a raisin and a grape? The raisin is a dehydrated grape. The next time you

13

want to skip out on your water intake think about the extra calories you will consume or remember what a wrinkled grape looks like because of the lack of water content. I think you will choose to drink the water.

How Much Water Should I Drink?

You may have heard "drink your 8 glasses of water", right? There is no scientific evidence that you should drink 8 glasses of water but a good rule of thumb is to drink half your weight in ounces.[7] If you're an athlete or have a strenuous job that causes the loss of lots of fluid it would be a good idea to drink extra water.

2. Fruits - "Nature's Candy"

If you are not eating fruit, there are many good reasons why you should, according to Harvard School of Public Health. Fruits have lots of vitamins and **antioxidants**. Anti-oxidants are believed to be the scavengers that gobble up the free radicals that are responsible for oxidation, aging and disease.

Antioxidants are substances found in many fruits that may protect cells from the damage caused by unstable molecules known as free radicals. It is believed that free radical damage may lead to cancer. Antioxidants interact with free radicals, stabilize them and may prevent some of the free radical damage. Some examples of antioxidants are beta-carotene, lycopene, vitamins A, E and C. [8]

Fruits have been found to help with preventing cancer, heart disease, blood pressure, and stroke as well as with digestive disorders.[9] Adding fruit to your daily dietary intake is good for you especially if you crave sugary snacks. Fruit is best eaten alone or with some healthy fats like nuts or seeds, to avoid the insulin spikes from the sugar.

Among the recommendations I make with my clients is 2-3 servings of fruit a day. It's best to choose fruits with a lower glycemic index.

What Is The Glycemic Index?

The glycemic index lists foods according to how they affect blood sugar. Eating foods that are high in the glycemic index will spike blood sugar levels, which over a period of time can lead to loss of sensitivity to **insulin** also known as insulin resistance. Insulin is a hormone that allows blood sugar to enter cells to be used as fuel for energy. When it's not used it stores the surplus as fat and over works the pancreas. Insulin is one of the hormones that contributes to weight gain and belly fat. Insulin resistance has been linked to diabetes, obesity and high blood pressure.

Which Fruits Are Best To Eat?

I encourage clients to eat fruits that have a lower glycemic index versus the higher glycemic index (GI) as noted in the chart below. Low GI is 0-55, Mid GI is 55-69, High GI is 70-100.[10] Fruits with a low glycemic index of 0-55 are the best choices with occasional consumption of fruits with a higher glycemic index of 70-100, due to their ability to stimulate blood sugar spikes.

Glycemic Index Range:
    Low = Less than 55
    Medium = 55 – 70
    High = More than 70

FRUIT	GLYCEMIC INDEX	SERVING SIZE
APPLE	38	4.5 ounces
APRICOTS	57	4.5 ounces
BANANAS	54	4.5 ounces
CANTALOUPE	65	4.5 ounces
CHERRIES	22	4.5 ounces
GRAPEFRUIT	25	4.5 ounces
GRAPES	46	4.5 ounces
HONEYDEW MELON	65	8.0 ounces
KIWI	53	4.5 ounces
MANGOS	56	4.5 ounces
ORANGES	44	4.5 ounces
PAPAYA	59	4.5 ounces
PEACHES	42	4.5 ounces
PEARS	38	4.5 ounces

PINEAPPLE	66	4.5 ounces
PLUMS	39	4.5 ounces
RAISINS	64	2.0 ounces
STRAWBERRIES	40	4.5 ounces
WATERMELON	72	4.5 ounces

3. Veggies – Nutrient Dense Food Vital For Your Health

Eating vegetables is essential for an overall healthful diet that may reduce the risk for many health conditions including heart disease and cancer. There are so many benefits to eating vegetables including:

- low in calories
- low in fat
- rich in fiber
- no cholesterol
- great source for potassium
- create a feeling of fullness which helps prevent overeating
- rich in Vitamin A & C, Folic Acid
- may help reduce blood cholesterol levels

If eating vegetables has not been part of your lifestyle, a good place to start is with leafy green vegetables. Start with adding a salad at lunchtime, mixed with bell peppers, carrots, broccoli, cucumbers, celery and tomatoes with oil and vinegar.

The Benefits Of Cruciferous Vegetables

The best vegetables for belly fat and promising studies of their anti-cancerous effects [11] are cruciferous vegetables. Cruciferous vegetables contain vitamins, minerals and glucosinolates, which are phytochemicals that help the body create its own natural antioxidant system also known as Phase II enzymes. They stimulate the liver to make detoxifying enzymes that block the free radical attack on DNA.[12]

Some of the most popular cruciferous vegetables are:

- Bok Choy
- Broccoli
- Brussels Sprout
- Cabbage
- Cauliflower
- Chinese Cabbage
- Collard Green
- Kohlrabi
- Mustard Green
- Rapini
- Rutabaga
- Turnip

Vegetables Are Low In Glycemic Index

Vegetables are highly nutrient dense foods that are great for regaining your health, weight loss and vitality. Most vegetables are low in the glycemic index and are loaded with vitamins! In the chart below you will find the *standard size* instead of the serving size, which typically indicates that the food has an insignificant amount of carbohydrates that would impact the blood sugar levels.

VEGETABLE	GLYCEMIC INDEX	SERVING SIZE
ARTICHOKES	15	Standard size
ASPARAGUS	15	Standard size
BEET	64	2 $\frac{4}{5}$ ounces
ROCCOLI	15	Standard size
CARROT (raw)	45	2 $\frac{4}{5}$ ounces
CAULIFLOWER	15	Standard size
CELERY	15	Standard size
CUCUMBER	15	Standard size
EGG PLANTS	15	Standard size
GREEN BEANS	15	Standard size
LETTUCE	15	Standard size
PARSNIPS	97	2 $\frac{4}{5}$ ounces
PEPPERS (all varieties)	15	Standard size
POTATO (baked)	85	5 $\frac{1}{4}$ ounces
POTATO (instant)	83	5 $\frac{1}{4}$ ounces
POTATO (steam)	65	5 $\frac{1}{4}$ ounces
POTATO (sweet)	54	5 $\frac{1}{4}$ ounces
SNOW PEAS	15	Standard size
SPINACH	15	Standard size
SUMMER SQUASH	15	Standard size
TOMATOES	15	Standard size
YAMS	51	5 $\frac{1}{4}$ ounces
ZUCHINI	15	Standard size

4.   Protein – Power Food

What Is Protein?

Protein is the basic building block of essentially every tissue of the body. Protein is made of 20 different amino acids. The human body can produce some of the amino acids and the remainder we get from the food we consume. Adequate protein is necessary for strength, development of muscle and increased athletic performance. Protein is also important for healthy hair, strong nails, beautiful skin and rebuilding tissues in your body. Most of your organs, muscles and hormones are made of protein.

Foods High In Protein

Most animal products are high in protein but they can also be high in cholesterol. Choose animal products that are organic, free range, grass fed, hormone free, antibiotic free and were raised in a humane way. Fish is another great source of protein with healthy fats. Eggs are a great source of easily digestible protein. Some of the foods that are high in protein include chicken, turkey, lamb, bison, beef, fish and eggs. Most animal products are high in protein but other sources of protein to consider are nuts, seeds, beans and grains.

Do Vegetables Have Protein?

Vegetables are great sources of vitamin and minerals but have a low protein content. If you are a vegetarian it's important to get protein from beans, nuts and seeds. A few of the high protein vegetables include asparagus, broccoli, cauliflower, okra and spinach.

5. Grains – The Good, The Bad and The Ugly

Any food that is made from wheat, oats, rye, barely and corn is considered a grain. [13] There are grains that are gluten free and grains that contain gluten. Gluten is a protein in grains. Some people have Celiac Disease, which is an autoimmune condition and consuming gluten causes their bodies to attack and damage the small intestine.

Grains with Gluten	Gluten-free Grains
• Barley • Oats** • Rye • Triticale • Wheat including durum, faro, kamut, spelt; others include bulgur, semolina	• Amaranth • Buckwheat • Millet • Quinoa • Rice • Sorghum • Teff • Wild Rice

[14]Table modified from "The Whole Grain Council"

** Depending on the source some classify oats as a gluten, because they are usually contaminated during the wheat growing process.

The Truth About Grains

I have to admit that I do enjoy eating gluten free grains like rice and quinoa but I must also say they really are not necessary in our diets. We have been lead to believe that grains have lots of fiber, in deed they do but so do fruits and vegetables and they are more easily digestible than grains.

Why Grains May Be Bad For You?

Grains contain lectins, which are proteins and are also found in some seeds, beans and potatoes. Lectins are not easily broken down and are resistant to digestive enzymes and hydrochloric acid (stomach acid). Lectins may create damage to the gut lining because they bind to the wall of the gut. Lectins can cross through the body via a damaged gut wall and bind to cell membranes, arteries, organs and glands. [15] They can create imbalance in the gastrointestinal system, which can lead to dysfunction and can lead to conditions as IBS, Celiac Sprue, Chron's Disease and degenerative diseases.

Should I Eliminate Grains?

There are different sources that will encourage elimination of all grains, some sources encourage elimination of grains with gluten, and some permit only amaranth, buckwheat, and quinoa as part of a healthy eating plan. Many people around the world have experienced relief of digestion issues, inflammation, joint pain, fatigue and chronic conditions with the elimination of grains.

The bottom line is to take personal responsibility for your health. If you eat foods that create digestive issues, pain, inflammation or any other symptoms then **don't have it.** Eliminate it from your diet and heal your gut and if you are curious then try it after 12 months and see what happens.

6. Fats – Necessary For Healthy Bodies

Back in the 80's the latest craze was to eliminate fat from the diet. The fat-free craze was born and so were numerous health problems. Fats are essential for a healthy body. We need fat for energy, healthy cell membranes and healthy nerve tissues. Some fats are more healthful than others. A low fat diet can be dangerous, and you will discover why our body needs fat.

Why Do I Need Fat In My Diet?

Our bodies need fat for many reasons:

- Healthy hormone production
- Healthy immune system
- Help keep you full
- Provide energy as a back up after blood sugar supplies are dry
- Help absorb vitamins
- Help with less cravings because it stays in the stomach longer
- May help with production of feel good hormones (endorphins)
- Needed for insulation support of organs, bones, nerve fibers, skin from cold and heat
- Helpful for healthy skin, hair and nails
- Helpful for inflammation

We need about 30% of our calories from fat which could be from 45-65 grams of fat per day depending on your caloric intake.

Types of Fat

There are different types of fat and some are better for you than others. Elimination of fat from your diet would not be a good choice and your health would suffer. You need fats for creating a healthy body but you must know which type of fat you should consume. Let's clear up the confusion as to which fats are to be avoided at all costs and which fats are necessary for promoting good health.[16]

Healthful Fats – Monounsaturated Fats & Polyunsaturated Fats

The best sources of fat are unsaturated fats founds in oils, nuts, seeds, and avocadoes. Other good sources of fat to include in your diet are fatty fish like salmon, tuna, trout, sardines, mackerel, and herring.

Unsaturated Fats are liquids at room temperature. They come mostly from plants. Monounsaturated fat and polyunsaturated fats are types of unsaturated fat.

Monounsaturated Fat	Polyunsaturated Fats
Vegetable oils (canola, olive, peanut) May help increase "Good" HDL cholesterol May lower risk of heart disease	Vegetable oils (safflower, sesame, sunflower) Mostly in seafood May lower "Bad" LDL cholesterol Types are Omega 3 and Omega 6 fatty acids

Unhealthful Fats - Saturated Fats & Trans Fats

Saturated fats are solid at room temperature. They are found mostly in animal products, such as milk, cheese, and meat. Saturated fat raises the low density lipoprotein (LDL) and the total cholesterol levels and can increase the risk for type 2 diabetes.

Poultry and fish have less saturated fat than red meat. Most of the saturated fat is also in tropical oils, such as coconut oil, palm oil, and cocoa butter. Foods made with butter, margarine, or shortening (cakes, cookies, and other desserts) have a lot of saturated fat. Saturated fats can raise your cholesterol. Minimize the consumption of saturated fats from beef, lamb, pork, chicken, and dairy products.

Eliminate all trans fats like those found in candy bars, margarine, shortening, prepackaged snack foods (microwave popcorn, cracker, chips), fried foods, non-dairy foods, like coffee creamer and whipped toppings. Most commercial baked pastries like doughnuts, muffins, cakes, cookies and pizza crust are loaded with trans fats and should also be avoided.

There are many types of fat but if you follow the guidelines above it should help you create a healthier lifestyle. Remember don't go NO-FAT but instead choose GOOD FAT.

Oils for Cooking and Salads

Coconut oil and almond oil are the best to cook with and to sauté vegetables in; olive oil is the best to drizzle over cooked foods or as a salad dressing with balsamic vinegar.

CHAPTER 3

Why Should I Juice?

Juicing has been one of the most superior and quickest methods to increase vitality, shed unwanted pounds, and to regain and optimize your health.

Meet Adequate Fruit and Veggie Requirements

According to the Center for Disease Control, a 44 year old female, with a physical activity level of 30-60 minutes a day should consume at least 2 cups of fruit and 2.5 cups of vegetables daily. The requirement for a 44 year old male, with a physical activity level of 30-60 minutes a day should consume 2 cups of fruit and 3.5 cups of vegetables daily. More aggressive practitioners recommend 7 servings of fruit and vegetables for women and 9 servings for men.

Other sources recommend 1 pound of fruits and vegetables for every 50 pounds of body weight. E.g. a 150 pound person should consume at least 3 pounds of fruits and vegetables. Dr. Eric Berg, the author of *The Seven Principles of Fat Burning* recommends eating 1/3 cup of fruit for every 1 cup of vegetables consumed. In other words the more vegetables you eat the more fruit you are allowed. I personally like the idea of eating 1 pound of vegetables for every 50 pounds of body weight and 1 serving of fruit for every pound of vegetable consumed.

Get Your Phytonutrients to Promote Vitality

Phytonutrients are organic compounds of plants that promote human health. Since phytonutrients are found in fruits and vegetables, it makes sense to eat foods that are rich in phytonutrients.

According to Dr. Frank Lipman phytonutrients[17]:

- Serve as antioxidants
- Are anti-inflammatory
- May help prevent cancer
- May help prevent heart disease
- Have anti-aging affects
- Enhance immune response
- Alter estrogen metabolism

A Living Organism Needs Live Food

Since you are a living organism that has a frequency, what better way to keep your body alive? Have you ever noticed what fish in the ocean eat? They eat live plants in the ocean. That's how they stay alive. Aren't you a beautiful living individual? Doesn't it make sense that to stay alert, vibrant, ageless, fit and healthy, a large percentage of your daily food intake should be raw food?

Why Should I Juice?

Healthy people have lots of *biophotons*. A biophoton is light emitting from the cells of living organisms. In other words it's light energy. Living plants get their light from the sun therefore have lots of biophotons. Raw juices have an abundance of light energy or biophotons, which allow you to have extraordinarily high energy. When you consume just 1 glass of fresh juice you are getting high performance food to supercharge your body with energy!!

Juice Fasting For Spiritual Clarity And Creativity

In the new and old testament of the bible, fasting is mentioned as a means to get one's focus off of material things including food, to focus on God and to improve mental, emotional and spiritual clarity. *Fasting* means abstaining from all or specific types of food and drink. Various fasts were practiced at that time, including abstaining from food, restriction of certain foods, abstaining from food and water. I wouldn't recommend the latter. Juice fasting has been found to be superior to water fast because you are supplying your body with densely packed nutrients for immediate energy!

Many people choose to fast for health reasons. The most common reason I find that people want to do a juice fast is to reboot their system for more energy, cleanse their bodies, and shed a few pounds. One of the benefits of a juice fast has also been a more focused and clear mind. Most people will use a juice fast as a means to making it a permanent lifestyle change for consuming more fresh fruits and vegetables.

Juice Fasting For Weight Loss

Many actors and entertainers who have to look and feel their absolute best in a short period of time and be able to keep up with the demands of 12-18 hour work days use juice fasting as their secret weapon. Janet Jackson, Ben Affleck, supermodel Christy Turlington and Liv Tyler are no strangers to the amazing benefits of juice fasting.

During a juice fast most people don't have a desire to eat processed foods because of the concentrated amounts of nutrients in the juice that allows them to feel energetic and prevents them from snacking on sugary and processed foods.

Juice Fasting For Vitality

I have personally juiced for years and one of the major benefits I have experienced is extraordinary health, mental clarity, energy and zest for life. These are some of the most common reasons people want to start juicing. When a person begins to experience low energy and their lack of drive for life has been exhausted, they begin to look for solutions to regain their vitality.

When you begin to ingest food that is nutrient dense, easily assimilated and absorbed, it results in extraordinary energy and vitality! It's a wonderful way for the body to utilize nature's finest food that is nutrient packed and ready for use. It's like switching from regular gas to premium gas for a sports car, the car runs more efficiently, is quicker and it's get up and go is much more smooth with the high octane premium gas.

The Secret to Anti-Aging

This is probably my favorite part of the book because living in Southern California where vanity is rampant and plastic surgery and Botox is the norm, I am pleased to say that I have not had either one. I remember when I was looking for a medical facility to integrate my alternative health practice in, the doctor's first words were "My gosh you look so young and healthy". Everything inside of me was jumping for joy saying, "Yes and thanks to a healthy lifestyle of juicing and eating chemical free food", while I simply smiled and said thank you.

There are lots of promises of anti aging creams, chemical peels, and scrubs that are suppose to make you look younger. But what really is important is what you put in your body not on

31

your body to make you look younger. Your skin is the largest organ of the body and what you put in your body affects your liver, kidneys and the added stress of detoxification. I remember sitting in a class and the instructor had one of the student's remove her make up for the sake of a demonstration and when she removed the makeup her skin was blotchy and unhealthy looking but you couldn't tell with the layers of toxic makeup covering up her blemishes. Our skin is exposed to lots of free radicals ranging from makeup, lotion, perfumes, laundry detergent, etc.

There is an increase in environmental toxicity that is contributing to the increase in disease and the accelerated aging process. What I love about juicing is the high content of vegetables and fruits that are loaded with antioxidants[18] which can help slow down the aging process by getting rid of free radicals from the skin that may cause premature aging. If the ladies spent as much money on fruits, vegetables and a good juicer as they do on anti-aging creams, they would look and feel better, as well as even shedding some of the extra weight that's making them look older.

Give Your Digestive System a Break from Processing Food

During a juice fast your digestive tract gets a rest. The energy needed to digest food is used to heal your body during the time of a fast. The digestive tract has been over worked from years of eating processed foods, foods with antibiotics, hormones, pesticides, fungicides and herbicides. It also allows your body to suppress the bad bacteria in the gut and feed the good bacteria. It will help improve gut flora (most depression and autoimmune conditions improve with juicing because it improves the gut flora which is important in developing a healthy immune system.)

Healing can occur during this time because most of the body's energy is used to digest food and remove toxins that can be harmful to the body. Most of us are toxic from the inside and may display it in our body externally in the form of acne, lifeless hair, weak nails, and sagging skin.

A Great Way to Get Instant Nutrition

The bottom line is that juicing is an easy and economical way to consume large amounts of vitamins, minerals, antioxidants, and enzymes to enhance your immune system and boost your energy!! It's like putting high performance gas in your car. I like to think of my green drinks as coffee on steroids, without the chemicals and with longer lasting effects and health benefits. The great benefit of fresh homemade juice is that your body knows what to do with it and you begin to feel the benefits right away!

~JUICING~

CHAPTER 4

What Should I Expect From Juicing?

Change in Energy Level

When I started juicing I felt the difference in my energy level immediately. Most people feel the same way because they are adding high-octane fuel (the fresh juice) to their car (their body). What kind of car do you want to be? Would you like to be a high performance sports car or a jalopy that stalls out and stops a lot?

❖ Action Step

What is your energy like now on a 0-10 scale (1= low and 10=incredible)?

_____

_____

_____

_____

How is this affecting your life?

_____

_____

_____

_____

Where would you like your energy level to be?

_____

_____

_____

_____

How would it change your life if you had
extraordinarily high energy? What things could
you to do that you are not doing now or that are
holding you back from doing them now because
of your health?

_____

_____

_____

_____

Rejuvenation of Your Cells

One of the wonderful benefits of adding fresh
juices to your current diet is that it offers your
body an abundance of nutrients.   It's like
someone depositing a million dollars in your
bank account. The fresh raw juices offer your
body a handful of nutrients to help it heal more
quickly and completely. Fresh juices offer a
super concentrated cocktail of power packed
nutrients that your body needs for repair,

rejuvenation, and helping to remove irritating toxic substances that contribute to disease and aging.

I believe the digestive tract gets the most benefit because the digestive system takes a break when you fast for at least 3-5 days and allow the epithelial cells to be replaced with healthy ones.

Major Benefits to be Gained

- Increase energy
- Increase stamina
- Rejuvenate your cells
- Improve mental clarity and mood
- Less mucus
- Better sleep
- Younger looking skin
- Shiny hair
- Stronger nails
- Flatter tummy
- Weight loss
- Decrease aches and pains
- Restore alkalinity
- Enable cell walls to return to their ideal state
- Cleanse the body
- Decrease inflammation
- Decrease acid reflux
- More focused concentration
- Increase confidence
- Alleviate allergies
- Regulate your body's pH

~JUICING~

CHAPTER 5

What Is The Difference Between Juice Fasting, Blending And Adding Juicing To My Current Dietary Regimen?

What is Juicing?

Many people choose to add more nutrients to their diet by adding 1-2 glasses of fresh juice to their daily regime. Juicing has been implemented as part of a healthy lifestyle by providing the body with the extracted juice from fresh fruits and vegetables that are high in vital nutrients that are easily assimilated. They find that the additional nutrients and vitamins fill them up and they eat less processed food. Most processed foods have very little nutritional value, never satisfying your appetite and leaving you hungry all the time.

Juice Fasting

A juice fast is a type of detox, which involves the intake of raw fruit and vegetable juice, and water for a predetermined time frame. Meals and snacks are replaced with raw fruit and raw vegetable juices. During this time no solid food is consumed. Juice fasting can be very beneficial but should be done properly and with the guidance of a practitioner.

Many people choose to do a 24-hour juice fast after they have added juice to their daily regime for at least one month. Once a 24-hour juice fast is completed they experiment with a 3-day juice fast and gradually work up to either a week or 30 days.

What is Blending?

One of the biggest mistakes I see is calling blending, "juicing". They are 2 totally different concepts. Blending is placing fruits and vegetables in a blender and consuming the juice and the pulp/fiber. It's a simple way to get your fruits and vegetables in your diet; it takes less time and it's easier to clean up. There are benefits to blending because it allows people to add more fruits and vegetables to their diet.

Adding It to Your Current Health Plan

Many people ask me if they should juice or blend. I tell them do both along with a healthy diet and exercise. If you start adding more fruits and vegetables to your diet by either juicing or blending, it's more than what you were eating before. Once your body gets accustomed to the new live food packed with super nutrients it may be time to consider a 24-hour juice fast.

CHAPTER 6

Steps For Getting Started!

#1 Have a Made Up Mind!

Decide on what you want out of your health and do it. It's that simple! No excuses. *I can't because I am going through a divorce, I have a deadline to meet, I don't have time, I have kids,* etc. If you don't take action now then when will you do it? The perfect time is NOW because something will always come up (wedding, baby shower, graduation, funeral, vacation, job hunting). Decide to be a better you and have better health.

- Do you want to have more energy?
- Do you want to feel better?
- Do you want to look better?
- Do you want to shed a few extra pounds?
- Do you want a clearer mind?
- Do you want to stop making excuses for why you can't do it?

Today is the time to start, so that you can have great health and vitality to do the activities you enjoy today and tomorrow!!

❖ Action Step

Decide whether you want to add juicing to your daily routine or 2-3 days a week. Maybe you would like to do a juice fast. Which type of fast would you like to do? You can choose a 24 hour fast, 3 day fast, 7 day fast, 10 day fast, 14 day fast or a 30 day fast?

_____

_____

_____

_____

Why that many days?

_____

_____

_____

_____

_____

_____

#2 Goals: What Does Great Health Look Like To You?

If you were planning a trip to Europe for 4 weeks, would you just pack your bags and go? Of course not, you would have to plan your trip, right? Most people would research the places they want to visit and plan their days in order to get the most out of their trip. The trip is only 30 days and most people go about their usual schedule when they return. My point is...they planned for a 30-day adventure and had alternatives available if their trip didn't work out exactly as planned.

Let's start planning and goal setting for the next few days. It doesn't matter if it is a 24 hour fast, a 30 day fast or if you want to add juicing to your eating plan for 30 days in order to experience the amazing results from juicing. You must know the end result before you start the journey. Let's plan it, in order to get the results you want.

❖ Action Step

What benefit do you hope to achieve? Be specific; is it more energy, better sleep, mental clarity, weight loss, beautiful skin and hair, to look younger?

_____

_____

_____

_____

_____

_____

❖ Action Step

Visualize yourself as a healthy, vibrant and fit person. What does that look like to you? Be very descriptive from the size of your waist, body fat percentage, tone of your skin, energy level. (E.g. I see myself as vibrant, exuding energy, shiny hair, 15% body fat, size 6, 8, 10, toned and sculpted legs, back and shoulders, radiant skin etc.) Be specific it's your body and you're the sculptor of the magnificent physique you are designing!

_____

_____

_____

_____

_____

_____

_____

❖ Action Step

Now that you have decided how many days you are going to fast, think about how you are going to reach your goal. Do you *plan* to buy a juicer or do you plan on purchasing fresh made juices from your local health food store or juice bar? If you plan on buying and what may be best for you. a juicer we will be educating you on the types of juicers available

_____

_____

_____

_____

_____

_____

❖ Action Step

If you are working long hours and planning a trip during the time of your fast, you will have to anticipate the possibilities that may arise and prepare for them. If you anticipate some long days at the office, now is the time to *plan* for them. I do not recommend bottled juices from the store. The juice is usually pasteurized and high in sugar. Purchase fresh juices from the local health food store or juice bar. Juice enough for 2 days and store them in amber colored bottles or stainless steel thermos to prevent rapid oxidation.

_____

_____

_____

_____

_____

_____

_____

_____

_____

_____

_____

#3 Buddy Up and Be Accountable

The top 3 reasons most people don't reach their goals is because they *don't plan*, they *don't visualize* themselves reaching their goals, and they don't have an *accountability partner*.

In Napoleon Hill's book "Think and Grow Rich" he mentions that successful people have a mastermind group/accountability group. Employees have employers they are accountable to, just like athletes have coaches who guide them and bring the best out in them.

When I see clients in the office or consult with them, I usually ask them, "What will be your consequences if you don't meet the goal at the end of the month?" Most people don't like to give their hard earned money away, so I ask them to put a monetary value on not sticking to the daily goal that will attain the results of the big goal at the end of the month. For example if they skip their workout and don't eat enough veggies for the day, they will have to put $3, $4, $5, or $10 in an envelope. At the end of the week, they give the envelope to a person whom is difficult to be around. Can you imagine giving your hard earned money to your foe because you didn't follow through with your commitment? Just thinking about that makes me cringe. Goals are most often not met; due to lack of accountability and consequences.

❖ Action Step

Who is going to be your accountability partner? Choose someone who will not let you off easy and will remind you of your desired outcome.

_____

_____

_____

_____

❖ Action Step

What will you tell them to keep you
accountable? E.g. remind you how you are
going to feel when you are no longer in pain,
remind you of the increased vitality and energy
you will have, the smaller and tighter body you
will get as the result of your accomplishment.
Write down what you want them to tell you and
how they can encourage you to stay on track.
They can't help you if they don't know what the
end result is, right?

_____

_____

_____

_____

_____

_____

_____

_____

❖ Action Step

Keep a food journal. Write down what you are eating and drinking, plus the quantities while on your mission to great health and a new body. This will help you stay accountable to yourself and discover what foods may provoke an allergic reaction.

_____

_____

_____

_____

_____

_____

_____

_____

_____

_____

_____

_____

❖ Action Step

If you don't have a person to support you then become part of our coaching program. I have several coaches in my own life who keep me accountable. What would you expect from us?

Be detailed and specific. Contact us now at
info@drlindamarquez.com and let us know you
want to become part of our coaching program.

_____

_____

_____

_____

_____

#4 Choosing a Juicer

When starting a juice fast, a blender is not an
option unless you buy cheesecloth to remove the
fiber. I don't prefer this method because of the
high oxidation that occurs during blending.
Remember the juice without the fiber allows
instant nutrition to your cells for quick
absorption and energy.

There are many juicers on the market that vary
in price range and quality. I believe you should
invest in what your budget will allow and one
that you will use. But I also believe that if you
are seeking permanent changes it is best to
invest in a juicer that will have a longer life
span. There are basically **3 types of juicers:**
centrifugal, masticating and auger/squeeze and
press.

Centrifugal Juicer

The centrifugal juicer is the most common juicer that is purchased when a person starts to add juicing into their lifestyle. The fruit and vegetables come in contact with a shredder type disc and the juice will exit through a spout and the pulp will be ejected from another spout into a canister on the opposite side of the juicer. Some don't have a spout and you have to remove the pulp from the main unit after about a quart of juice is collected. It's best to choose a juicer with an ejection spout for the pulp.

Cost: $30 - $200

Pros: Easy to use, easy to clean and a great first time investment

Cons: Will not last as long as a masticating juicer, less nutrient value than a masticating juicer, less juice extraction from fruits and vegetables

Brand Names: Breville Juicers, Juiceman Juicer, Jack Lalane, Omega, L'Equip, Waring

Masticating Juicer

The masticating juicers "masticate" or chew the fruit and vegetables to extract the juice. It uses an auger with "teeth" type blades to squeeze the remaining contents.

Cost: $260- $350

Pros: Versatile, durable, quieter, makes nut butters, baby foods, desserts, juices wheat grass, easy to use and clean

Cons: Bulkier, heavier than and not as attractive as the centrifugal type, slow juicer

Brand Names: Champion, Lexen, L'Equip, Omega, Samson

Auger Juicer

The auger type juicers are becoming popular. The augers rotate at low revolutions per minute allowing for higher yield content and nutrient content. They are either single or double augers, which squeeze and press the fruits and vegetables.

Cost: $230- $400

Pros: More juice is extracted and is preferred by raw food enthusiasts because of the higher nutrient yield; it makes nut butters, baby foods, desserts, juices wheat grass and is easy to use and clean

Cons: More expensive, slower, larger and heavier than other juicers, longer cleaning time

Brand Names: Greenstar, Omega 8000 series, Samson Multi-purpose

❖ Action Step

If juicing is going to be part of your lifestyle, which I hope it will be, I would invest in a masticating or Auger juicer. If you are short on countertop space a centrifugal juicer may work best for you. If you plan on adding wheat grass into your diet and have a family, then the masticating juicer may be best for you. If you are a raw food enthusiast the auger juicer is a good fit. Choose a juicer you will use and let's get moving!

_____

_____

_____

_____

~JUICING~

NOTES:

_____

_____

_____

_____

_____

_____

_____

_____

_____

_____

_____

_____

_____

_____

_____

_____

_____

CHAPTER 7

Taking Action For A Juice Fast And Permanent Lifestyle Changes

Wake Up Your Taste Buds

This is the 2nd most exciting part of the process. There are many fruits and vegetables that you have never tasted that have amazing health benefits. This is the time to wake up your taste buds and excite them with nature's food. Most of us have perverted taste buds that thrive on sugar, artificial sweeteners, man made chemicals, and processed foods that have destroyed our health.

Choose Organic Fruits and Vegetables

In order to get the healthiest juice, choose organic fruits and vegetables. Look for the "certified organic" labels and the #9 on the labels of fruits and vegetables. By choosing organic fruits and vegetables you are avoiding the billions of pounds of pesticides and herbicides that are sprayed on our crops yearly. [19] These pesticides and herbicides pose short and long term health risks including but not limited to nerve damage, tremors, vomiting, convulsions, cancer, and birth defects. Always purchase *organic* fruits that are listed below, because non-organics are heavily sprayed with harmful chemicals.[20]

- Apples
- Blueberries
- Grapes
- Nectarines
- Peaches
- Strawberries

If you are on a budget and need to skimp on buying organic, the fruits listed below have minimal or no pesticides.

- Avocado
- Cantaloupe
- Grapefruit
- Kiwi
- Mangoes
- Pineapple
- Watermelon

Choose fruits and vegetables that are in season. Avoid fruits and vegetables that are wilted, moldy, over ripened or that have brown spots.

Juice, Primarily Vegetables

The biggest mistake most first time juicers make is they consume a lot of fruit juice and very little vegetable juice. The suggested proportion is 70-80% vegetables and 20-30% fruits. It is best to choose organic vegetables for juicing. There are vegetables that are heavily sprayed with chemicals so you want to make sure you buy organic.

Listed below are the **highly contaminated** vegetables with pesticides and herbicides.[22]

- Celery
- Collard Greens
- Kale
- Lettuce
- Potatoes
- Spinach
- Sweet Bell Peppers

I highly encourage you to purchase all organic produce because I don't want you consuming juice (or fuel for your body) that is contaminated. There are a few vegetables that have the **least contamination** and exposure to pesticides, as listed below.[22]

- Asparagus
- Cabbage
- Eggplant
- Mushrooms
- Onion
- Sweet Corn
- Sweet Peas
- Sweet Potatoes

It is best to consume juice after it has been prepared to get the maximum antioxidants.

~JUICING~

Choosing Vegetables and Fruits for Juicing

If you're new to juicing, start with the first 3 steps. The following measurements will yield about 12 to 20 ounces in a masticating juicer and less in a centrifugal juicer. Adjust the amount according your taste buds and the desired amount.

Step #1

- Apple (1-2)
- Carrots (1)

These vegetables are not as dense as some of the other green vegetables.

Add one or two of the following vegetables:

Step #2
- Celery Stalks (2-3)
- Cucumber (1)
- Spinach (2-3 bunches)
- Endive (1/2 head)
- Green Leaf Lettuce (6-7 leaves)
- Red Leaf Lettuce (6-7 leaves)
- Romaine Lettuce (6-7 leaves)
- Escarole (1 cup chopped)

Step #3 Add one to two of the following fruits:

- Apples (1)
- Cranberries (1/2 cup)
- Lemons (1) (they do an amazing job cutting out the green taste)
- Limes (1)

Step #4 Add one of the following (1/2 to 1 head):

- Bok Choy
- Cabbage (Red, Green, Nappa, Savoy)

Step #5 Add a bitter vegetable (1-2 leaves)

- Kale
- Collard Greens
- Dandelion Greens
- Mustard Greens

Step #6 Add herbs (small handful):

- Cilantro
- Ginger (some times categorized under spices) ½ to 1 inch*
- Parsley
- Fennel

A little bit of ginger goes a long way and gives your juice a "little kick"

These are only guidelines for the beginner. I recommend that you start with the vegetables you enjoy eating; start with those and add one of the fruits mentioned. I also enjoy adding carrots for their beta carotene (be careful because of their high sugar content), which may not be suitable for diabetics. Another favorite to add is a few chunks of pineapple. They contain bromelain, a proteolytic enzyme that helps digest protein, and also has anti-inflammatory benefits. Experiment with different types of fruits and vegetables. Be careful with grapefruits since they can intensify the action of medications. Soft fruits such as berries, bananas, avocadoes are not ideal for juicing but are great for raw soups.

If you are new to juicing, drinking more than 8 ounces of green drink at one time may be too strong for your body. Green juices are like mixed cocktails; you should sip on them throughout the day. If you have been juicing for a few weeks and want strength, green juices are the way to go.

❖ Action Step

Take the 1st step and start with you favorite fruits and vegetables. What are some of your favorite fruits and vegetables you can juice?

Taking Action

Fruits:

_____

_____

_____

_____

Vegetables:

_____

_____

_____

_____

Juice fasting has helped me to get healthy, stay fit, strengthen my immune system, look younger, feel better, and improve my mind and clarity. These amazing benefits can be obtained if you follow the guidelines in this book.

~JUICING~

NOTES:

_____

_____

_____

_____

_____

_____

_____

_____

_____

_____

_____

_____

_____

_____

_____

_____

_____

_____

CHAPTER 8

Getting The Most Out Of A Juice Fast

What Do You Want From a Juice Fast?

Do you see yourself healthier, more energetic, and slimmer with vibrant skin? Successful people see themselves and act as if they have already reached their goals. They carry a 3x5 card in their wallet, on their iPod, iPhone, sticky notes on their computer, on their mirrors, in their bathrooms, in their cars and remind themselves daily of the person they want to become. You are successful otherwise you wouldn't be taking the steps to do this!

❖ Action Step

Get a 3x5 card and write your health goals on it. Carry it with you and read it at least 2 times a day, upon arising in the morning, before going to bed and many times throughout the day. Write it on the space below as a reminder in case you misplace your card.

_____

_____

_____

_____

How Do You Want to See Yourself?

When we start something we need to know what
the end results are going to be. If you plan a trip
to the beach on a hot day, you know that you
will be going in the ocean to cool off and enjoy
your day. You can see your day unfold, before it
even happens. Take your health a step forward
and have a visual of what that looks like to you.
Every successful person I have known has a
vision board. A vision board is a tool used to
help clarify, and help you focus on a specific
goal. *A vision board is any type of board
(poster, white, cork), on which you can display
images and words that represent whatever you
want to be, have or do in your life.* It is your
ideal life before your eyes.

❖ Action Step

Take the time to sit for a minute and see the new
you. Who do you see? Gather pictures of the
new you and start your vision board today.

_____

_____

_____

_____

_____

_____

Attitude of Gratitude

I have many patients who journal daily about what they are eating but also about what they are grateful for in their lives. Keep a small notebook and write 3 things before you go to bed that you were grateful for on that day. Maybe it was making a new friend, having clean water, having two eyes, a loving family or a job. We can always find something to be grateful for, even when we have had a challenging day.

❖ Action Step

_____

_____

_____

_____

_____

_____

_____

_____

_____

Prepping For a Fast

The biggest mistake I have seen and personally experienced is eating the wrong foods before a fast, whether it's a 24 hour fast or 30 day fast. Sometimes we go in with the mindset, "I am going to fast for 24 hours (or whatever you choose), and so I am going to pig out before I start. This is the wrong mindset when you are preparing for a juice fast or any dietary changes for a healthier body. Below you will find some guidelines to help you get the maximal benefits from a juice fast.

- Add organic fruits and vegetables to your current diet.
- Add one glass of fresh juice to your current dietary regime on the 7th and 6th days prior to starting your fast, and 2 glasses of organic fresh juice on the 5th, 4th and 3rd days prior to your fast, add 2-3 glasses of organic fresh juice the 2 days prior to starting your fast.
- Eliminate or taper off sugar, dairy, animal products, caffeine, fried and processed foods one week prior to your fast.
- Increase your water intake to at least ½ your body weight in ounces.
- Eat less and avoid overstuffing yourself.

Getting The Most Out Of A Juice Fast

* The most effective method I have experienced and seen with extended and short term juice fasts is eating salads, slightly steamed vegetables, fruit, legumes, less than 25 grams of chicken, turkey or fish prior to a fast.

What to Do During a Fast

Stay focused on the benefits you will be experiencing when you complete the fast. See your vision board daily and review your goals on your 3X5 card.

- Drink water - Drink at least ½ half your body weight in ounces
- Get some sunshine throughout the day, 20-30 minutes
- Walk outdoors (intense exercise is not recommended for beginners)
- Get 7-8 hours of uninterrupted sleep

Coming Off of a Fast

The second biggest mistake I have seen when people come off a fast is they eat the wrong foods. Almost all the benefits of a juice fast are lost because of this mistake.

Below is a general guideline for breaking a fast the right way.

~JUICING~

Day #1

Continue drinking juice and add 2 pieces of fruit. Divide each piece of fruit in half and consume 4 servings.

Day #2

Drink fresh juice and food from day 1

Add lightly steamed non-starchy vegetables, such as spinach, broccoli, cauliflower, cabbage, brussel sprouts, asparagus, artichoke, and squash

Day #3

Drink fresh juice and foods from days 1 & 2

Add organic eggs from grass fed chickens or wild caught fish and a fresh salad

Day #4

Drink fresh juice and foods from day 1, 2 & 3

Add organic chicken or poultry and a fresh salad

Day #5

Drink fresh juice and foods from days 1, 2, 3 & 4

Add brown rice and a fresh salad

Day #6

Drink fresh juice and foods from days 1, 2, 3, 4 & 5

Add beans and gluten free grains. Avoid wheat, oats, rye, barley and corn. Oats are inherently gluten free but are frequently contaminated with wheat during the growing or processing methods. There are several companies that offer pure and uncontaminated oats (Bob's Red Mill, Cream Hill estates, GF Harvest, Avena Foods, Legacy Valley, and Gifts of Nature).

Gluten free grains include amaranth, buckwheat, millet, montina (Indian Rice Grass), quinoa, sorghum, teff, rice and wild rice.

Day #7

Add other wholesome foods, as desired

When introducing foods back into the diet follow these guidelines:

- Avoid overeating
- Chew food slowly
- Note any reactions such as bloating, gas, diarrhea, constipation, lethargy, skin reactions or other symptoms from the foods you are re-introducing back into your eating plan
- Transition into a new lifestyle change of eating more healthful raw food and

chemical free foods as a long term eating plan, which would include avoiding processed foods, fried foods, sugary laden foods and gluten (if you have tested positive to gluten)

Adding Exercise to Maximize Your Health

One of the fastest ways to reap the benefits for your new found journey to great health is by adding exercise to your new regime, if you are not exercising at the time.

One of the best exercises for an extended juice fast is walking and yoga, because of the improved circulation and breathing. These two improved functions allow more oxygenation of the blood cells. Other more strenuous exercises are best done once you have completed several juice fasts and you have become familiar with how your body reacts during a juice fast.

Take the Next Step to Extraordinary Health

When I talk to people or clients I ask them, when was the last time they had their blood work up done. Almost all of them say never or it's been at least a couple of years. I believe everyone needs to know what their current health status is. A person without symptoms is not necessarily healthy. Do you know anyone who has had a stroke, heart attack, or cancer while appearing to be healthy because they did not have any symptoms or they ignored them? Blood tests will show your current health status, and also screen for any underlying conditions that may prevent you from reaching your health goals.

There are millions of people who have diabetes, cardiovascular disease, cancer, anemia, and compromised immune systems who are about to die any day. Juicing, taking vitamins, and eating wholesome foods are great ways to regain your health but you first have to know where you are and what systems in your body need immediate attention.

I like to share my story because I believe it is relevant to why blood tests are important. I am a wellness educator, author and in private practice, yet my own health was failing and this was discovered via blood, saliva tests and other diagnostic tests. This scenario is very common among health care practitioners. Without these tests I would not be enjoying my life nor be able to share my personal experience with thousands of people about how to regain their health. Unfortunately most doctors are as sick as their patients and do not take the steps for improving their own health.

Take the next step in optimizing your health. Diagnostic tests are one of the best ways to see where your baseline health is and to determine a starting point for future comparison. We will be glad to assist you with this process. Email us at info@drlindamarquez.com, with "Blood Tests" in the subject heading.

Putting It Altogether and Taking Action

- Prepare mentally for the days you have chosen to fast.
- Prepare at least 7 days before an extended juice fast by consuming only organic fruits, organic vegetables and organic legumes (beans, nuts and seeds). Eliminate or drastically reduce animal products, processed foods, sugar, alcohol, dairy products, nicotine, grains, and eggs. An ideal diet during the preparation phase should be 70-80% raw fruits, vegetables, legumes and 20-30% of the food mentioned above.
- The best time to fast is during the warmer months of the year, late spring, summer and early fall.
- It's important to drink plenty of water (half your weight in ounces).
- Use organic fruits and vegetables during the fast.
- Drink between 50 ounces and 80 ounces of juice daily.
- A combination of fruits and vegetables should be used (70-80% vegetables and 20-30% fruit) for preparation of juices.
- Incorporate exercise outdoors to increase circulation and oxygen to the cells.

Walking and/or yoga are great exercises for the beginner.
- Focus on your outcome – vision board, journaling.

NOTES FOR JOURNALING:

_____

_____

_____

_____

_____

_____

_____

_____

_____

_____

_____

_____

_____

_____

_____

_____

CHAPTER 9

Juice Recipes For Extraordinary Health

The recipes in this chapter yield 8-12 ounces, approximately 1 serving, unless otherwise noted. Slowly add one vegetable or fruit at a time in the juicer. Juice the softer fruits or vegetables (pineapple or cucumber) first, followed by a more firm fruit or vegetable (apple or celery).

ABC Juice

2 apples
4 carrots
2 beets
6 kale leaves or 1.5 cups
1.5 inch piece of ginger

Cut the ingredients to easily fit into the feeder tube of your juicer. Put them through the mouth of the juicer one ingredient at a time. Juice the ingredients. Pour them into a tall glass, stir, drink as soon as possible and enjoy!

Serving 1

Adrenal Booster

3 carrots
2 kale leaves
1 handful of parsley
2 celery stalks
1 tomato
1 lemon
Dash of cayenne pepper
Dash of sea salt

Put all the fruit and vegetables through the mouth of the juicer one ingredient at a time. Pour into a large glass, add cayenne pepper and sea salt, then stir.

Servings 1 -2

Anti-inflammatory Rejuvenator

5 carrots
1 cup pineapple chunks
½ cup of dark leafy greens of your choice (kale, spinach)
1 inch ginger root

Cut the ingredients to easily fit into the feeder tube of your juicer. Put them through the mouth of the juicer one ingredient at a time. Juice the ingredients. Pour them into a tall glass, stir, drink as soon as possible and enjoy!

Servings 1 -2

Apple Lemonade

1 green apple
2 cups of kale
2 cups of spinach
4 celery stalks
½ cucumber
1 small lemon

Cut the ingredients to easily fit into the feeder tube of your juicer. Put them through the mouth of the juicer one ingredient at a time. Juice the ingredients. Pour them into a tall glass, stir, drink as soon as possible and enjoy!

Serving 1

Afternoon Delight

4-6 carrots
4-6 stalks celery
2 roma tomatoes
1/2 bunch cilantro
1 lemon

Cut the ingredients to easily fit into the feeder tube of your juicer. Put them through the mouth of the juicer one ingredient at a time. Juice the ingredients. Pour them into a tall glass, stir, drink as soon as possible and enjoy!

Serving 1

Apple Celery Surprise

2 green apples
4 celery stalks
1 small cucumber
2 cups of spinach
2 cups of kale
1.5 inch piece of ginger

Cut the ingredients to easily fit into the feeder tube of your juicer. Put them through the mouth of the juicer one ingredient at a time. Juice the ingredients. Pour them into a tall glass, stir, drink as soon as possible and enjoy!

Serving 1

Apple Green Rejuvenator

1 pink lady apple
1 lemon
2 kale leaves
1 cucumber
1 celery stalk
1 inch of ginger

Cut ingredients to easily fit into the feeder tube of your juicer. Put ingredients through the mouth of the juicer one at a time. Juice the ingredients. Pour into a tall glass, stir, drink as soon as possible and enjoy!

Serving 1

Arthritis Reliever

2 carrots
½ cucumber
1 cup of kale
1 cup of spinach
½ green apple
1 inch piece of ginger

Cut the ingredients to easily fit into the feeder tube of your juicer. Put them through the mouth of the juicer one ingredient at a time. Juice the ingredients. Pour into a tall glass, stir, drink as soon as possible. Enjoy!

Serving 1

Blackberry Surprise

2 pears
3 celery stalks
3 carrots
3 kale leaves
1 bunch of parsley
1 cup of blackberries

Put all the fruit and vegetables through the mouth of the juicer one ingredient at a time. Pour into a large glass and enjoy.

Add some water and a drop of stevia, a natural sweetener, if you want to dilute the juice a bit. Enjoy!

Serving 1

Beauty Skin Express

2 cucumbers
1 carrot
½ red bell pepper
½ green apple

Cut the ingredients to easily fit into the feeder tube of your juicer. Put them through the mouth of the juicer one ingredient at a time. Juice the ingredients. Pour them into a tall glass, stir, drink as soon as possible and enjoy!

Serving 1

Blood Builder

1 beet
1 cucumber
1 handful of dandelion greens
1 lemon
2 carrots

Cut the ingredients to easily fit into the feeder tube of your juicer. Put them through the mouth of the juicer one ingredient at a time. Juice the ingredients. Pour them into a tall glass, stir, drink as soon as possible and enjoy!

Serving 1

Brocco Express

2 cups of kale
¼ head of green cabbage
2 broccoli stalks
1 green granny apple
½ lemon
1/2 inch piece of ginger root

Cut the ingredients to easily fit into the feeder tube of your juicer. Put them through the mouth of the juicer one ingredient at a time. Juice the ingredients. Pour into a tall glass, stir, drink as soon as possible. Enjoy!

Serving 1

Chilling Cucumber Cilantro

1 cucumber
2 stalks of celery
2 leaves of bok choy
2 green kale leaves
2 carrots
2 sprigs of mint
2 sprigs of cilantro
1 lime

Cut the ingredients to easily fit in the feeder tube of your juicer. Juice the ingredients. Pour them into a tall glass, stir, drink as soon as possible and enjoy!

Serving 1

Cranberry Delight

1 red apple
½ cup frozen cranberries
½ lemon, peeled
½ beet root

Cut the ingredients to easily fit into the feeder tube of your juicer. Put them through the mouth of the juicer one ingredient at a time. Juice the ingredients. Pour them into a tall glass, stir, drink as soon as possible and enjoy!

Serving 1

Cravings Rescuer

3-4 large kale leaves
1 whole stalk of leek
1 lemon
1 large tomato
1/2 bunch cilantro
3-4 carrots
½ inch piece of ginger

Cut the ingredients to easily fit into the feeder tube of your juicer. Put them through the mouth of the juicer one ingredient at a time. Juice the ingredients. Pour them into a tall glass, stir, drink as soon as possible and enjoy!

Serving 1

Extreme Power House Drink

1 lemon
2 cups of alfalfa sprout
½ -1 inch piece of fresh ginger
2 carrots
3 cucumbers
1/2 bunch parsley

Cut the ingredients to easily fit into the feeder tube of your juicer. Put them through the mouth of the juicer one ingredient at a time. Juice the ingredients. Pour them into a tall glass, stir, drink as soon as possible and enjoy!

Serving 1

Forever Young

4 carrots
1 cucumber
1 lemon
½ yellow bell pepper

Cut the ingredients to easily fit into the feeder tube of your juicer. Put them through the mouth of the juicer one ingredient at a time. Juice the ingredients. Pour them into a tall glass, stir, drink as soon as possible and enjoy!

Serving 1

Ginger Surprise

1 inch piece of ginger
6 carrots
1 lemon
1 apple

Cut the ingredients to easily fit into the feeder tube of your juicer. Put them through the mouth of the juicer one ingredient at a time. Juice the ingredients. Pour them into a tall glass, stir, drink as soon as possible and enjoy!

Serving 1

Goddess of Greens

3-4 leaves of kale
5 large romaine lettuce leaves
1 beet
1/2 bunch of cilantro
1 lemon
2 cups fresh spinach
1/2 apple

Cut the ingredients to easily fit into the feeder tube of your juicer. Put them through the mouth of the juicer one ingredient at a time. Juice the ingredients. Pour them into a tall glass, stir, drink as soon as possible and enjoy!

Serving 1

Grapefruit Surprise

1 large pink grapefruit, peeled
½ cup pineapple chunks
1 inch piece of ginger

Cut the ingredients to easily fit into the feeder tube of your juicer. Put them through the mouth of the juicer one ingredient at a time. Juice the ingredients. Pour them into a tall glass, stir, drink as soon as possible and enjoy!

Serving 1

Green Apple Delight

2 green apples
2 large carrots
¼ head of red cabbage
6 Swiss chard leaves
1 small lemon
1 inch piece of ginger

Cut the ingredients to easily fit into the feeder tube of your juicer. Put them through the mouth of the juicer one ingredient at a time. Juice the ingredients. Pour them into a tall glass, stir, drink as soon as possible and enjoy!

Serving 1

Green Detox Shock

½ green apple
1 large beet
3-4 leaves beet tops
3-4 carrots
3-4 celery stalks
¼ inch
1 lemon

Cut the ingredients to easily fit into the feeder tube of your juicer. Put them through the mouth of the juicer one ingredient at a time. Juice the ingredients. Pour into a tall glass, stir, drink as soon as possible. Enjoy!

Serving 1

Green Lemonade

1 head romaine lettuce or celery
5 to 6 stalks kale (any type)
1 to 2 apples (as needed for sweetness-Fuji's are a great choice)
1 whole organic lemon (don't peel it)
1-2 tablespoon fresh ginger (optional)

Cut the ingredients to easily fit into the feeder tube of your juicer. Put them through the mouth of the juicer one ingredient at a time. Juice the ingredients. Pour into a tall glass, stir, drink as soon as possible. Enjoy!

Serving 1

Green Sweet Surprise

½ of red cabbage
3-4 stalks celery
4 kale leaves
1 lemon
1 lime
1 apple
¼ inch piece of fresh ginger

Cut the ingredients to easily fit into the feeder tube of your juicer. Put them through the mouth of the juicer one ingredient at a time. Juice the ingredients. Pour them into a tall glass, stir, drink as soon as possible and enjoy!

Serving 1

Heart Helper

4 carrots
2 celery stalks
1 cucumber
2 garlic cloves
1 handful of parsley

Cut the ingredients to easily fit into the feeder tube of your juicer. Put them through the mouth of the juicer one ingredient at a time. Juice the ingredients. Pour them into a tall glass, stir, drink as soon as possible and enjoy!

Serving 1

Lemon Lime Delight

1 lemon
1 lime
2 Asian pears
2 granny smith apples
2 carrots
2 cups purple cabbage
1 ½ inch piece of ginger

Cut ingredients to easily fit into the feeder tube of your juicer. Put them through the mouth of the juicer one ingredient at a time. Juice the ingredients. Pour into a tall glass, stir, drink as soon as possible and enjoy!

Serving 1

Mighty Greens

2 granny smith apples
2 cups of spinach
6 leaves of Swiss chard
1 cucumber
4 celery stalks
½ medium fennel bulb
1 handful of basil
1 inch piece of ginger root

Cut ingredients to easily fit into the feeder tube of your juicer. Put them through the mouth of the juicer one ingredient at a time. Juice the ingredients. Pour them into a tall glass, stir, drink as soon as possible. Enjoy!

Serving 1

Mighty Green Machine

1 cucumber
4 celery stalks
2 granny smith apples
7 kale leaves
1 lemon
1 inch piece of ginger

Cut the ingredients to easily fit into the feeder tube of your juicer. Put them through the mouth of the juicer one ingredient at a time. Juice the ingredients. Pour them into a tall glass, stir, drink as soon as possible and enjoy!

Serving 1

Mint and Citrus Juice

2 oranges
2 celery stalks
1 carrot
½ pink grapefruit
¼ bunch of mint

Cut the ingredients to easily fit into the feeder tube of your juicer. Put them through the mouth of the juicer one ingredient at a time. Juice the ingredients. Pour them into a tall glass, stir, drink as soon as possible and enjoy!

Serving 1

Morning Sunshine

4 carrots
½ cup of spinach
2 kale leaves
2 stalks of celery
1 lemon
1 cucumber
1 inch of ginger root

Cut the ingredients to easily fit into the feeder tube of your juicer. Put them through the mouth of the juicer one ingredient at a time. Juice the ingredients. Pour them into a tall glass, stir, drink as soon as possible and enjoy!

Serving 1

Morning Riser

4-6 carrots
4 stalks of celery
1 lemon
1 Macintosh apple

Cut the ingredients to easily fit into the feeder tube of your juicer. Put them through the mouth of the juicer one ingredient at a time. Juice the ingredients. Pour them into a tall glass, stir, drink as soon as possible and enjoy!

Serving 1

Orange Morning Surprise

4 oranges
2 apples
4 celery stalks
2 lemons
1 cucumber
1 cup pineapple
2/3 cup cranberries

Cut the ingredients to easily fit into the feeder tube of your juicer. Put them through the mouth of the juicer one ingredient at a time. Juice the ingredients. Pour them into a tall glass, stir, drink as soon as possible and enjoy!

Serving 4

Pain & Cramp Reliever

2.5 ounces of spinach
½ of a medium size pineapple
1.5 inch piece of ginger
½ small fennel bulb

Cut the ingredients to easily fit into the feeder tube of your juicer. Put them through the mouth of the juicer one ingredient at a time. Juice the ingredients. Pour them into a tall glass, stir, drink as soon as possible and enjoy!

Serving 1

Potassium Booster

3 carrots
3 celery stalks
½ bunch parsley
½ handful of spinach

Cut the ingredients to easily fit into the feeder tube of your juicer. Put them through the mouth of the juicer one ingredient at a time. Juice the ingredients. Pour them into a tall glass, stir, drink as soon as possible and enjoy!

Serving 1

Reboot Juice (Inspired from the movie "Fat, Sick and Nearly Dead")

1 bunch of kale
4 celery stalks
1 cucumber
2 granny apples
½ lemon
½ inch piece of ginger root

Cut the ingredients to easily fit into the feeder tube of your juicer. Put them through the mouth of the juicer one ingredient at a time. Juice the ingredients. Pour into a tall glass, stir, drink as soon as possible. Enjoy!

Serving 1

Super Cleanser Delight

2-3 carrots
4 cucumbers
½ inch of fresh Ginger
1 lemon
1 beet

Cut the ingredients to easily fit into the feeder tube of your juicer. Put them through the mouth of the juicer one ingredient at a time. Juice the ingredients. Pour them into a tall glass, stir, drink as soon as possible and enjoy!

Serving 1

Summer Delight

2 white peaches
2 broccoli steaks
1 Fuji apple

Cut the ingredients to easily fit into the feeder tube of your juicer. Put them through the mouth of the juicer one ingredient at a time. Juice the ingredients. Pour them into a tall glass, stir, drink as soon as possible and enjoy!

Serving 1

Super Green Elixir

2 stalks of swiss chard
1 green apple
2 stalks of celery
1 cucumber
A handful of parsley

Cut the ingredients to easily fit into the feeder tube of your juicer. Put them through the mouth of the juicer one ingredient at a time. Juice the ingredients. Pour them into a tall glass, stir, drink as soon as possible and enjoy!

Serving 1

Super Workout Drink

1/2 romaine lettuce
3-4 leaves of kale
3-4 carrots
1/2 bunch carrot top
1 apple
1 lime

Cut the ingredients to easily fit into the feeder tube of your juicer. Put them through the mouth of the juicer one ingredient at a time. Juice the ingredients. Pour them into a tall glass, stir, drink as soon as possible and enjoy!

Serving 1

Sweet Delight

1 lime
1 large tomato
2-3 carrots
2 cups fresh spinach
1/2 carrot top bunch
1/2 bunch parsley
1 stalk of celery

Cut ingredients to easily fit into the feeder tube of your juicer. Put them through the mouth of the juicer one ingredient at a time. Juice the ingredients. Pour them into a tall glass, stir, drink as soon as possible. Enjoy!

Serving 1

Vitality Green Drink

1 large cucumber
6 celery stalks
1 apple
1 lemon
1 handful of spinach
1 handful of dandelion greens
1-inch piece of ginger

Cut ingredients to easily fit into the feeder tube of your juicer. Put them through the mouth of the juicer one ingredient at a time. Juice the ingredients. Pour into a tall glass, stir, drink as soon as possible and enjoy!

Serving 1

Weight Loss Booster

4 carrots
1 small Jerusalem artichoke
1 small beet

Cut the ingredients to easily fit into the feeder tube of your juicer. Put them through the mouth of the juicer one ingredient at a time. Juice the ingredients. Pour them into a tall glass, stir, drink as soon as possible and enjoy!

Serving 1

CHAPTER 10

Awesome Blended Smoothies, Drinks And Soups

The following recipes in this section are not juices but can be introduced when preparing for a juice fast or when breaking a juice fast. The following recipes require a high speed blender. I prefer the Vitamix. *See Appendix A for recommended blenders.*

You will also note some of the recipes call for protein powders for additional nutritional support. *See Appendix B for recommended protein powders.*

Awesome Smoothies & Blended Drinks

California Cocktail Smoothie

½ cup of coconut milk
1 teaspoon of organic vanilla
¼ teaspoon of cinnamon
4-5 drops of *Sweet Leaf Vanilla Crème Stevia Drops*
1 frozen banana
1 cup frozen strawberries
2-3 ice cubes

Blend all ingredients and serve.

Serving 1

~JUICING~

California Green Smoothie

½ cup coconut milk
¼ avocado
½ cup spinach
½ banana, frozen
1 tablespoon raw honey
1-2 ice cubes

Freeze spinach for about 1- 1 ½ hours

Place all the ingredients in a blender. Blend until creamy and smooth. Serve immediately

Serving 1

Chocolate Peanut Butter Protein Smoothie

2 cups of coconut milk or almond milk
1 scoop of *Paradise Orac-Energy Protein & Greens* (or protein powder of your choice)
1 teaspoon *Chatfield's All Natural Cocoa Powder*
1 frozen banana
4-5 drops of *Sweet Leaf Chocolate Raspberry Stevia Drops*
2 tablespoons of peanut butter
5-6 ice cubes

Blend all ingredients and serve.

Servings 2

Dr. Linda's Colonade - (*helps detoxify the body and helps elimination*)

1 celery stalk
1 bunch of parsley
½ teaspoon olive oil
Juice of a medium to a large lemon

Place ingredients in blender and blend for about 1 minute. Drink immediately or sip on it throughout the morning or afternoon and enjoy.

Drink juice 2 times a day (upon rising and before dinner) for 2 weeks. After the first 2 weeks, drink every other day.

Serving 1

Green Smoothie

2 cups of leafy greens (kale, parsley, spinach)
1 cup of berries (blueberries, strawberries, raspberries, or cranberries)
½ cup of unsweetened coconut milk
½ frozen banana

Place ingredients in blender and blend for about 1 minute. Drink immediately or sip on it throughout the morning or afternoon and enjoy.

Servings approximately 1-2

Natural Colon Cleanse Juice

1 medium to large piece of cactus
Juice of 2 lemons
1 stalk of celery
1 garlic clove
½ slice of pineapple
2 pieces of parsley
½ cup of distilled or purified water or 4 ice cubes
1 small piece of aloe vera

Place ingredients in the blender and blend for about 1 minute. Drink immediately or sip on it throughout the morning. This special blend will help your skin and revitalize you. This is a morning drink.

Options: add cayenne pepper for taste, add 2 tablespoon of pine nuts after blending.

Serving approximately 4

Power Sports Drink

Most sports drinks are loaded with high fructose corn syrup, sugar, dyes and chemicals that cause liver dysfunction, metabolic syndrome and obesity. Here is a healthy inexpensive alternative that can be customized for your taste buds!

1 liter of clean filtered water or kangen water (Dasani and Aquafina are the worst bottled waters)
½ tsp. baking soda
½ tsp. sea salt
2 tbsp. of agave nectar or coconut sugar
2 tbsp. of unsweetened orange juice, pomegranate juice or lemon juice

Mix all ingredients in a bottle.

*Optional 1/4 Potassium Compound Powder

Sip on it as you would a sports drink.

Serving 4

Sunrise Strawberry Energy Smoothie

1 cup frozen organic strawberries
½ cup coconut milk
1 scoop of *Paradise Orac-Energy Protein & Greens* or any other plant based protein powder (see recommended list in appendix)
4-5 drops of Sweet Leaf chocolate raspberry stevia drops
1 tablespoon of *Natural Factors Rx Omega-3 Factors EPA 1,500 mg/DHA 750 mg*
1 tablespoon of *Vita-Myr Peruvian Inca Gold Maca*
1 tablespoon of Chia seeds
3-4 ice cubes

Place strawberries, coconut milk, and stevia into a blender (preferably a Vitamix) and blend. Place the remainder of the ingredients one at a time and blend, except the ice cubes. Add one ice cube at a time and blend until smooth and the desired consistency. Pour in tall glass or container

Note: If your smoothie is too thick add more milk and blend to desired consistency.

Serving 1

Super Greens Drink

1 cup organic caffeine-free green tea or
purified water
2 large kale leaves
1 cup spinach
½ orange without the skin
1 kiwi
1 small banana

Place ingredients in blender and blend for
about 1 minute. Drink immediately or sip on it
throughout the morning or afternoon. Enjoy.

Serving 1

Supreme Green Optimizer Drink

3 cups organic caffeine-free green tea
4 cups (loosely packed) of spinach or kale
2 apples
1 lemon (peeled)
1-3 cups of water for desired consistency

(Optional):
½ cup of frozen berries or
¼ tsp. of powder stevia or
½ cup of organic coconut sugar
1 scoop *Paradise Orac-Energy Protein &
Greens*

Place ingredients in blender and blend for
about 1 minute. Drink immediately or sip on it
throughout the morning or afternoon. Enjoy.

Servings approximately 3-4

Wrinkle Fighter Smoothie

1 cup frozen organic
blueberries/strawberries
½ cup spinach
½ cup coconut milk
1 scoop of *Paradise Orac Protein & Greens*
or any other plant based protein powder (see
recommended list in appendix)
4-5 drops of *Sweet Leaf Berry Stevia drops*
1 tablespoon of *Natural Factors Rx Omega-
3 Factors EPA 1,500 mg/DHA 750 mg*
5 drops *BioSil Advanced Collagen
Generator*
3-4 ice cubes

Place berries, coconut milk, and stevia in a
blender (preferably a Vitamix) and blend.
Blend in the remainder of the ingredients
one at a time except ice cubes. Add one ice
cube at a time and blend until smooth and to
the desired consistency. Pour in tall glass or
container and enjoy!

*Note: If your smoothie is too thick add more
milk and blend to desired consistency.*

Serving 1

Nutritious Raw Soup Recipes

<u>Creamy Bell Pepper Soup</u>

Ingredients:

2 medium sized red or yellow bell peppers, stems removed, chopped
2 medium cucumbers, chopped
½ medium red onion, chopped
¼ cup cold pressed olive oil from a dark bottle or coconut oil
1 teaspoon sea salt
1 teaspoon caraway seeds
2 medium cloves garlic
3 cups filtered water

Combine all the ingredients in a high-speed blender and blend until creamy and smooth.

Servings 8

Creamy Broccoli Soup

Ingredients:

2 - 3 cups of water
2 cups organic broccoli
1 large avocado
1 garlic clove
1 tablespoon grape seed or extra virgin olive oil
1 cup unsalted raw cashews
1 teaspoon chopped onions
1 teaspoon pink sea salt
1 teaspoon raw honey
¼ teaspoon cayenne or black pepper
¼ teaspoon cumin

Blend water, cashews, and broccoli until smooth. Add the rest of the ingredients and blend until creamy.

Servings 4

<u>Curry Carrot Soup</u>

6 carrots, chopped
1 ½ avocado
2 garlic cloves
1 lemon, peeled
2 teaspoon curry powder
1 teaspoon powdered ginger
¼ teaspoon cumin
Pinch of cayenne pepper
Dash of sea salt & black pepper to taste

Directions:

Toss all ingredients in blender and blend until smooth. For a pretty finish, sprinkle with curry powder.

Servings 4

Latin Gazpacho Soup

This is a quick soup that is tasty and only takes a few minutes to make. You will need a blender, a food processor would be great for chopping the vegetables but is not necessary. It takes about 20 minutes.

Ingredients:

¼ cup extra virgin olive oil
¼ cup lemon juice
5 large ripe tomatoes
2 cloves garlic or spicy pepper to taste
1 tablespoon raw honey or agave nectar
½ teaspoon sea salt
1 bunch fresh basil
1 medium bell pepper, cut into ¼ inch cubes
4 stalks celery, cut into ¼ inch cubes
1 large avocado, cut into ¼ inch cubes
1 small onion, cut into ¼ inch cubes
Chopped parsley

Directions:

Blend the olive oil, lemon juice, tomatoes, garlic, honey, sea salt and basil with ½ cup of water until smooth.

Pour the soup into a large bowl, and add the chopped avocado, bell pepper, celery and onion.

Mix all the ingredients together and sprinkle with chopped parsley.

Servings 4 - 5

Raw Spinach Soup

6 ounces of organic baby spinach leaves
1 cup water
1-2 cloves raw garlic
2 teaspoon of lemon juice
1 ripe avocado, cut in half and pitted
1-2 dates
¼ cup raw cashews salt to taste

Place all ingredients in a high-speed blender
like a Vitamix, for a few seconds until
you have a creamy consistency and add
water for a thinner consistency.

Servings 2

Spicy Spinach Soup

Ingredients:

3 small avocados (or one extra large)
2 small lemons, peeled and seeded
2 red or green bell peppers
½ bunch cilantro
3 cups of pure water
½ bunch organic spinach
½ teaspoon sea salt
1 small jalapeno pepper
Cabbage, Napa or red

Put all the ingredients in a high-speed blender like a Vita-Mix and blend well using the tamper. Once the ingredients are well blended, pour the soup into a large bowl.

Add thinly sliced Napa cabbage or red cabbage and dulse flakes or leaves. Enjoy!

Servings 6-7

CHAPTER 11

Q & A
Commonly Asked Questions About Juicing

Who Shouldn't Juice Fast?

- Pregnant and nursing moms
- The elderly
- Diabetics
- Growing children
- Hypoglycemics
- Underweight people
- Critically ill people
- People with kidney dysfunction

Every case is different and if you are uncertain whether you should fast, consult a qualified professional who is familiar with fasting and practices fasting.

Can I Use a Blender For Juicing?

No. A blender does not preserve the enzymatic value as much as juicing does and includes the pulp. I have heard of individual's blending and pouring the juice through a strainer and collecting it in container. I would not recommend this.

Can I Store The Juice?

It's best to consume them immediately after they are made or they can be stored up to 2 days. If you decide to store the juices for later consumption, take the precaution to store them properly. Fill a stainless steel thermos, dark amber bottle or mason jar to the top until it overflows and store immediately in the refrigerator. By overfilling the containers it minimizes oxidation of the juices.

Are The Bottled Store Juices Healthful?

Most bottled store juices are high in sugar and are pasteurized, which leads to the loss of their high potency nutrients.

Don't We Need the Fiber that is Lost During Juicing?

We definitely need fiber in our diets and should get it in our diets by eating vegetables and fruits. This book is for the purpose of obtaining extraordinary health in the quickest way possible. Juicing requires the least amount of effort for the absorption of nutrients.

Should I Dilute My Juice?

Dilution of juice is a personal preference. Some people like to dilute 50% of their juice with water.

What Are the Most Common Reasons People Juice?

The most common reasons for juicing is to increase the consumption of vegetables and fruits because of the high nutritional content and their antioxidant affects for fighting disease. Some other reasons include energy boost, immune system enhancement, weight loss, anti-aging, regulation of the body's pH and detoxification.

When is the Best Time to Drink Juice?

The best time to drink freshly juiced drinks is in the morning ½ hour before breakfast for optimum high nutrient absorption and in the afternoon for an energy boost.

How Much Juice Should I Drink?

If you are adding juicing as a way of life, start with one glass in the morning and add one in the afternoon after a couple of weeks. Many people drink juice when they are thirsty during a juice fast and consume about 50-80 ounces of juice during a 24 hour period. The key during a juice fast is to keep your appetite satisfied by sipping on juice throughout the day.

Do I have to Juice with Organic Fruits and Vegetables?

Organic is always preferred, otherwise you are getting a high dosage of toxins with your juices.

Which are the Best Vegetables to Juice?

The vegetables you will eat! Celery, cucumber and spinach are mild vegetables if you are new to juicing. Dandelion greens, parsley and wheat grass are great after you have acquired a taste for juicing.

Which are the Best Fruits to Juice?

Start with the fruits you enjoy like apples, oranges, grapes or watermelon. Most recipes use apples or carrots as their base for juicing and adding greens like cucumber, celery and spinach.

Which is the Best Juicer to Buy?

Most people will buy several juicers. If you are new to juicing the Jack Lalane Juicer or Breville Compact Juice Fountain Juicer would be a great start. The advantage of these two juicers is they remove the juice quickly from fruits and vegetables.

If you plan on making this part of your lifestyle I always recommend either an Omega or Champion juicer. They are masticating juicers, which yield a high juice content and retain most of their nutritional value even after 12 hours. The disadvantage is the cost and it takes longer to juice fruits and vegetables.

Are Fruit Juices Sugary?

Fruit juices do have a high content of natural sugar and are not recommended for diabetics or persons with Candida. As you will note in the recipe section of the book there are recipes that have mostly vegetables with some fruits that are tasty, even for the little ones.

Are There Some Vegetables and Fruit for Health Conditions?

Juicing fruits and vegetables yields a highly concentrated amount of anti-oxidants, which have been linked to anti-aging, vitality; and may even be affective against cancer and certain autoimmune conditions. Please see the list below.

Specialty Juice Blends

Anti-cholesterol or cholesterol fighter	Carrot, parsley, spinach, garlic
Anti-inflammatory or Inflammation fighter	Barley Grass juice powder
Anti-oxidant effects	Carrot, orange, green pepper, ginger
Arthritis	Greens, wheatgrass
Cold Eliminator	Carrot, lemon, ginger, radish, garlic
Detoxifier	Apple, beet, ginger, cucumber
Digestion Booster	Papaya, pineapple
Electrolyte Enhancer	Celery
Gallstones	Lemon
Headaches	Carrot, spinach, parsley, celery
Immune Enhancer	Carrot, celery, parsley, garlic
Liver Cleanser	Apple, beet, carrot, parsley
Liver Detoxifier	Wheatgrass
Memory Helper	Carrot, spinach, parsley, kale
Stress Helper	Carrot, celery, kale, spinach, dandelion greens

APPENDIX A

Recommended Blenders

Purchasing a quality blender is as important as the juicer you buy because you are transitioning into a new way of life and not a temporary diet. In the list below are some of the recommended blenders. Note that all blenders are not alike even from the same manufacturer, therefore stick to these recommended brands.

Vitamix TurboBlend 4500
Vitamix 1782 TurboBlend
Vitamix 5200
Breville Hemisphere Control BBL 605
Ninja Master Prep Pro QB1004
Kitchen Aid Model Number KSB5650MC 5-Speed Blender
Oster BCBG08-C 6 cup Glass jar 8-Speed Blender
Oster BCCG08-B2B 8 –Speed Blender
Cuisinart Smart Power CPB -300 (great for single servings and travelers)
Hamilton Beach Single Server Blender 51101B

APPENDIX B

Recommended Protein Powders

I strongly recommend adding a high quality plant based protein for those who want to add additional protein to their daily routine. In the list below are some of the recommended protein powders that are plant based and easy to digest.

Amazing Grass Amazing Meals Plain

Garden of Life Raw Protein
Garden of Life Raw Meal
Green Foods True Vitality
Jeff's Best Hemp Protein Powder
Living Harvest Hemp Protein
Paradise Protein & Greens
Vega Complete Whole Food Health Optimizer: Berry Flavor, Chocolate Flavor, Natural Flavor
Warrior Power Nutritionals Warrior Food The Ultimate Protein Supplement

NOTES:

1. http://www.cdc.gov/chronicdisease/over view/index.htm
2. http://www.cdc.gov/nchs/fastats/lcod.htm
3. http://www.naturalnews.com/009278.html
4. http://articles.mercola.com/sites/articles/ archive/2011/10/26/prescription-drugs-number-one-cause-preventable-death-in-us.aspx
5. Source: http://www.pbs.org/healthcarecrisis/ uninsured.html
   Article "Health Care Crises"
6. http://www.cms.gov/Research-Statistics-Data-and-Systems/Statistics-Trends-and-Reports/NationalHealthExpendData/ downloads/highlights.pdf
7. http://www.watercure.com/faq.html
8. http://www.cancer.gov/cancertopics/fact sheet/prevention/antioxidants
   Antioxidants and Cancer Prevention: Fact Sheet
9. http://www.hsph.harvard.edu/nutritionso urce/vegetables-full-story/
10. Lieberman, Shari (2006), *Glycemic Food Index Guide*. Garden City Park: Square One Publisher

11. http://www.cancer.gov/cancertopics/fact sheet/diet/cruciferous-vegetables
12. http://www.sharecare.com/question/gluc osinolates_protect_cancer
13. http://wholegrainscouncil.org, "Gluten Free Whole Grains"
14. http://wholegrainscouncil.org
15. http://www.naturaltherapypages.co m.au/article/Lectins, "What are lectins?"
16. http://www.mayoclinic.com/health/fat/N U00262, "Dietary Fats: Know which types to choose"
17. http://www.drfranklipman.com/what-are-phytonutrients/
18. http://www.huffingtonpost.com/2013/06/ 10/anti-aging-look-younger_n_3397282.html "Anti-Aging: 8 items That May Slow The Aging Process"
19 http://www.fda.gov/Food/FoodborneIlln essContaminants/Pesticides/UCM20067 97.htm Residue monitoring reports, 2009 Report & Data Base
20 http://www.ewg.org/foodnews/summary. php, EWG's 2013 Shopper's Guide to Pesticides in Produce

NOTES:

NOTES:

_____

_____

_____

_____

_____

_____

_____

_____

_____

_____

_____

_____

_____

_____

_____

_____

_____

_____

Made in the USA
San Bernardino, CA
17 February 2017